BREAKING FREE

FROM DIABETES

YOUR COMPLETE

GUIDE TO REVERSING

TYPE 2 DIABETES

DR. BELISA SAAVEDRA-KINNARD, PT, DPT

Dedication

In Memory of my dad, aka, Pops who instilled the love of God in us so that we would rejoice instead of weep in his final days. May you rest in Paradise until we meet again.

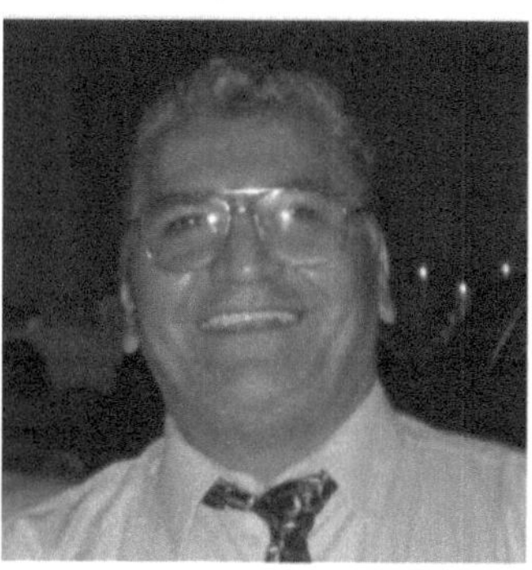

Special Thanks

I would like to thank my husband and my family who supported me throughout my life. Without their encouragement to pursue my PT career none of this would be possible today and to my sons Randell Jr and Micah whom are my driving forces to become a better person.

HEALTH ADVICE DISCLAIMER

The information contained in this report is not intended or implied to be a substitute for professional medical advice, diagnosis, or treatment. This report is intended to help the readers be better informed consumers of health care and is presented for general information/advice purposes only. Users of this guide are advised to do their own due diligence when it comes to their health decisions. Always consult your primary care professional for your individual needs.

The material in this guide may include information or products by third parties. Third Party Materials comprise of the products and opinions expressed by their owners. As such, I do not assume responsibility or liability for any Third Party material or opinions. By reading this report, you agree that myself and my company is not responsible for the success or failure of your health decisions relating to any information presented in this guide.

ABOUT THE AUTHOR

Dr. Belisa Saavedra-Kinnard

Dr. Belisa has been practicing Physical Therapy for the past ten years.

Her most recent decision to transition into treating patients with type2 diabetes was based on her own experience with gestational diabetes and the loss of her father to diabetes as well as hypertension (high blood pressure).

With an increasing prevalence of diabetes in her community, Dr. Belisa has made it her mission to help people beat type2 diabetes just as she did through proper nutrition and exercise for long term results.

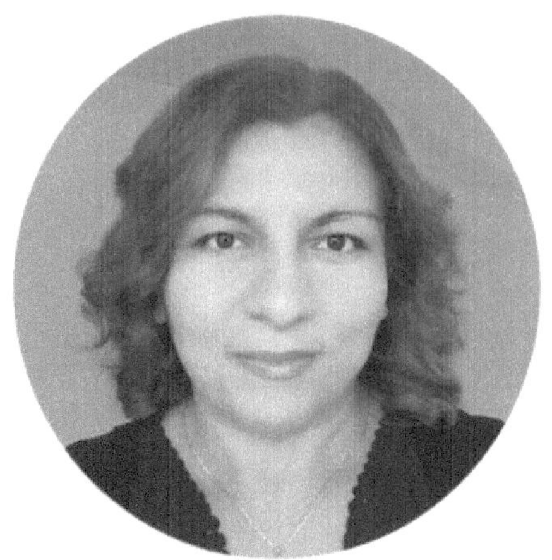

Table of Contents

Chapter 1

Risk Factors for Type 2 Diabetes

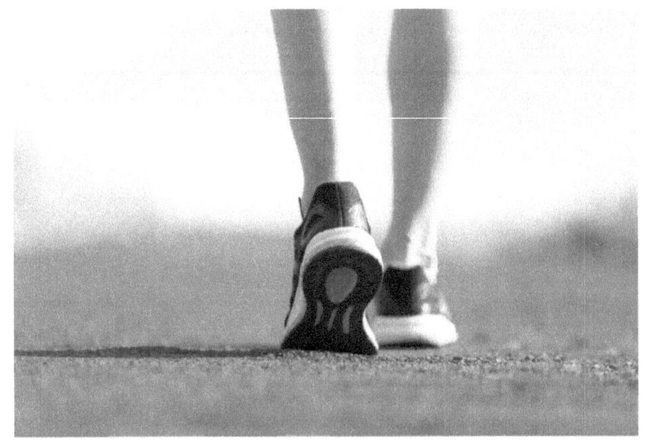

Risk Factors for Type 2 Diabetes

Did you know?

Diabetes affects around 30.3 million Americans, or about 9.4 percent of the U.S. population. Nearly 1 in 4 adults with diabetes, or 7.2 million Americans are unaware they even have the disease.

About 15 million women in the United States have diabetes. That's about 1 in 9 adult women.

However, another 84.1 million Americans have prediabetes, a condition which blood glucose levels are higher than normal, but not high enough to be diagnosed as diabetes.

9 out of 10 adults with prediabetes do not know they have it.
Here are the main risk factors:

Overweight or obesity: A Body mass index (BMI) of 25 or higher for adults.

Older age: 45 or older.

High blood pressure: Taking medicine for high blood pressure or having a blood pressure of 140/90 mmHg or higher.

High cholesterol: HDL cholesterol of 35 mg/dL or lower and triglycerides of 250 mg/dL or higher

Personal history of heart disease or stroke

Lack of physical activity: active less than three times a week.

Family health history: Having a mother, father, brother, or sister with diabetes

Race/ethnicity: Family background of African-American, American Indian/Alaska Native, Hispanic, Asian-American, and Native Hawaiian/Pacific Islander

Women have additional risks when:

Having a baby that weighed 9 pounds or more at birth Having diabetes during pregnancy (gestational diabetes) Having polycystic ovary syndrome (PCOS)

After menopause, women are at higher risk for weight gain, especially more weight around the waist, which raises the risk for type 2 diabetes

If you have any of these risk factors, talk to your doctor about ways to lower your risk for diabetes.

You can also take the Diabetes Risk Test and talk about the results with your doctor.

Other Complications From Diabetes

The extra glucose in the blood that leads to diabetes can damage your nerves and blood vessels. Nerve damage from diabetes can lead to pain or a permanent loss of feeling in your hands, feet, and other parts of your body.

Blood vessel damage from diabetes can also lead to:
Heart disease
Stroke
Blindness
Kidney failure
Leg or foot amputation
Hearing loss

Women with diabetes are also at higher risk for:
Problems getting pregnant

Problems during pregnancy, including possible health problems for you and your baby Repeated urinary and vaginal infections

Signs and Symptoms of Diabetes

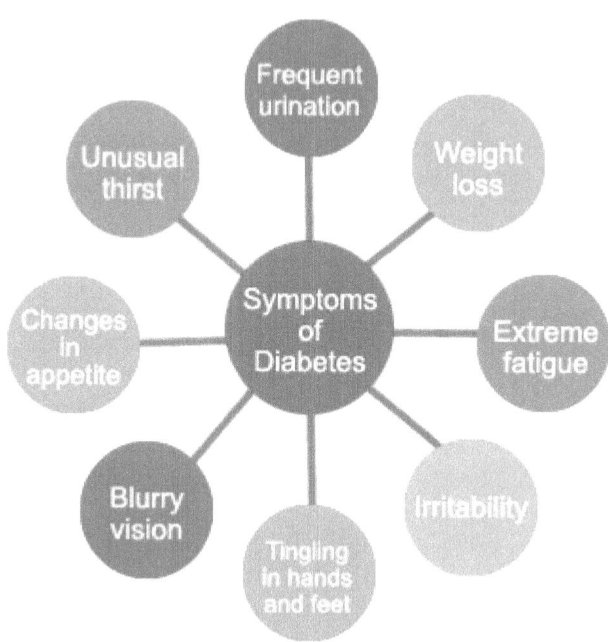

Chapter 2
Diagnosis and Treatment

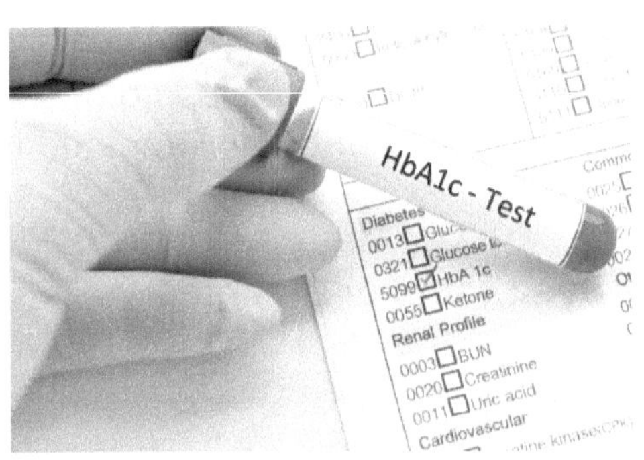

Diagnosis and Treatment

Your doctor will use a blood test called an A1C to see if you have diabetes. This test gives an average of your blood glucose over the last 3 months.
If the testing shows that your blood sugar levels are high (greater than 6.5), you can begin making healthy changes to your eating habits and getting more physical activity to help prevent diabetes.

Type 2 diabetes treatment may include taking medicine to control your blood sugar. Over time, people with type 2 diabetes make less and less of their own insulin. This may mean that you will need to increase your medicines or start taking insulin shots to keep your diabetes under control.

Weight Loss:

Treatment and Prevention

Studies have shown that you can prevent diabetes by losing weight. Weight loss through healthy eating and more physical activity improves the way your body uses insulin and glucose.
Obesity is a leading risk factor for diabetes. Calculate your BMI to see whether you're at a healthy weight. If you're overweight or obese, start making small changes to your eating habits and get more physical activity. Even a small amount of weight loss (7%, or about 14 pounds for a 200-pound woman) can delay or even prevent type 2 diabetes.

Eating healthy:

Treatment and Prevention

Choose vegetables, whole grains (such as whole wheat or rye bread, whole grain cereal, or brown rice), beans, and fruit. Read food labels to help you choose foods low in saturated fat, trans fat, and sodium. Limit processed foods and sugary foods and drinks.

Getting active:

Aim for 30 minutes of continuous physical activity consisting of both cardio and resistance training most days of the week and limit the amount of time you spend sitting.

Chapter 3
Meal Planning

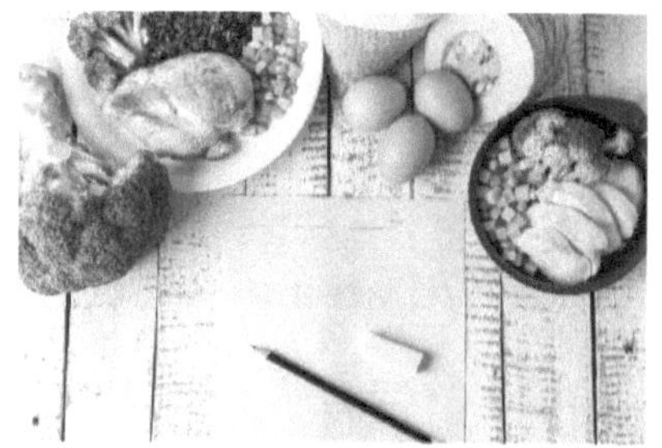

Meal Planning

Carbohydrate Counting for People with Diabetes

Counting carbohydrate servings may help you control your blood glucose level so that you feel better.

The balance between the carbohydrates you eat and insulin determines what your blood glucose level will be after eating.

Carbohydrate counting can also help you plan your meals.

Foods with carbohydrates include:

Breads, crackers, and cereals

Pasta, rice, and grains

Starchy vegetables, such as potatoes, corn, and peas
Beans and legumes

Milk, soy milk, and yogurt

Fruits and fruit juices

Sweets, such as cakes, cookies, ice cream, jam, and jelly

In diabetes meal planning, 1 serving of a food with carbohydrate has about 15 grams of carbohydrate:

Check serving sizes with measuring cups and spoons or a food scale.

Read the Nutrition Facts on food labels to find out how many grams of carbohydrate are in foods you eat.

The food lists in this handout show portions that have about 15 grams of carbohydrate.

An Eating Plan tells you how many carbohydrate servings to eat at your meals and snacks. For many adults, eating 3 to 5 servings of carbohydrate foods at each meal and 1 or 2 carbohydrate servings for each snack works well.

In a healthy daily Eating Plan, most carbohydrates come from:

At least 6 servings of fruits and nonstarchy vegetables

At least 6 servings of grains, beans, and starchy vegetables, with at least 3

servings from whole grains

At least 2 servings of milk or milk products

Check your blood glucose level regularly. It can tell you if you need to adjust when you eat carbohydrates.

Eating foods that have fiber, such as whole grains, and having very few salty foods is good for your health.

Eat 4 to 6 ounces of meat or other protein foods (such as soybean burgers) each day. Choose low-fat sources of protein, such as lean beef, lean pork, chicken, fish, low-fat cheese, or vegetarian foods such as soy. Eat some healthy fats, such as olive oil, canola oil, and nuts.

Eat very little saturated fats. These unhealthy fats are found in butter, cream, and high-fat meats, such as bacon and sausage.

Eat very little or no trans fats. These unhealthy fats are found in all foods that list "partially hydrogenated oil" as an ingredient.

The Nutrition Facts panel on a label lists the grams of total carbohydrate in 1 standard serving. The label's standard serving may be larger or smaller than 1 diabetic carbohydrate serving.

To figure out how many carbohydrate servings are in the food:

First, look at the label's standard serving size. Check the grams of total carbohydrate. This is the amount of carbohydrate in 1 standard serving. Divide the grams of total carbohydrate by 15. This number equals the number of carbohydrate servings in 1 standard serving. Remember: 1 carbohydrate serving is 15 grams of carbohydrate.

Note: You may ignore the grams of sugars on the Nutrition Facts panel because they are included in the grams of total carbohydrate.

1 serving=about 15 grams of carbohydrate

1 slice bread (1 ounce)

1 tortilla (6-inch size)

1⁄4 large bagel (1 ounce)

2 taco shells (5-inch size)

1⁄2 hamburger or hot dog bun (3⁄4 ounce) 3⁄4 cup ready-to-eat unsweetened cereal

1⁄2 cup cooked cereal

1 cup broth-based soup

4 to 6 small crackers

1/3 cup pasta or rice (cooked)

1⁄2 cup beans, peas, corn, sweet potatoes, winter squash, or mashed or boiled potatoes (cooked)

¼ large baked potato (3 ounces)

¾ ounce pretzels, potato chips, or tortilla chips

3 cups popcorn (popped)

1 small fresh fruit (¾ to 1 cup)

½ cup canned or frozen fruit

2 tablespoons dried fruit (blueberries, cherries, cranberries, mixed fruit, raisins)

17 small grapes (3 ounces) 1 cup melon or berries

½ cup unsweetened fruit juice

1 cup fat-free or reduced-fat milk

1 cup soy milk

2/3 cup (6 ounces) nonfat yogurt sweetened with sugar-free sweetener

2-inch square cake (unfrosted) 2 small cookies (2/3 ounce)

½ cup ice cream or frozen yogurt ¼ cup sherbet or sorbet

1 tablespoon syrup, jam, jelly, table sugar, or honey 2
tablespoons light syrup

Count 1 cup raw vegetables or 1⁄2 cup cooked
nonstarchy vegetables as zero (0) carbohydrate
servings or "free" foods. If you eat 3 or more servings
at one meal, count them as 1 carbohydrate serving.

Foods that have less than 20 calories in each serving
also may be counted as zero carbohydrate servings
or "free" foods.
Count 1 cup of casserole or other mixed foods as 2
carbohydrate serving

SAMPLE 1-DAY MENU FOR DIABETICS

Breakfast	1 extra-small banana (1 carbohydrate serving) 3/4 cup corn flakes (1 carbohydrate serving) 1 cup low-fat or fat-free milk (1 carbohydrate serving) 1 slice whole wheat bread (1 carbohydrate serving) 1 teaspoon margarine
Lunch	2 ounces turkey slices 2 slices whole wheat bread (2 carbohydrate servings) 2 lettuce leaves 4 celery sticks 4 carrot sticks 1 medium apple (1 carbohydrate serving) 1 cup low-fat or fat-free milk (1 carbohydrate serving)
Afternoon Snack	2 tablespoons raisins (1 carbohydrate serving) 3/4 ounce unsalted mini pretzels (1 carbohydrate serving)
Evening Meal	3 ounces lean roast beef 1/2 large baked potato (2 carbohydrate servings) 1 tablespoon reduced-fat sour cream 1/2 cup green beans 1 cup vegetable salad 1 tablespoon light salad dressing 1 whole wheat dinner roll (1 carbohydrate serving) 1 teaspoon margarine 1 cup melon balls (1 carbohydrate serving)
Evening Snack	6 ounces low-fat sugar-free fruit yogurt (1 carbohydrate serving) 2 tablespoons unsalted nuts

Chapter 4
Got H20?

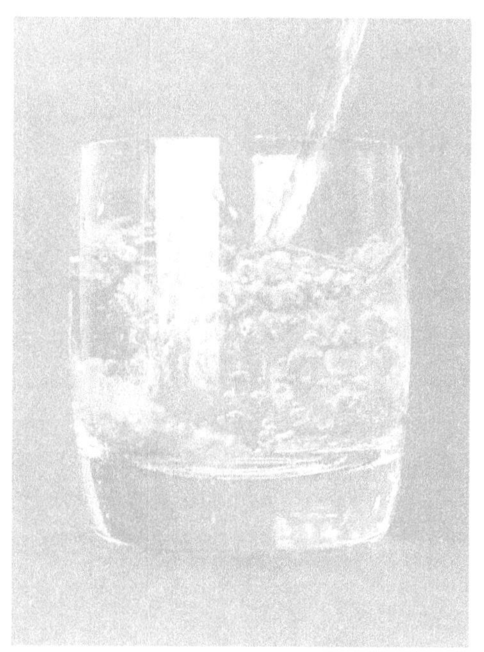

Got H2O?

H2O also known as water. Did you know our bodies are made up of 60% water? This is why it's so important to make sure you are getting enough of it every day. Replacing sugary drinks with water helps decrease your blood sugar spikes.

There are so many benefits to drinking enough water. In the follow graphic you will see a few of the important ones.

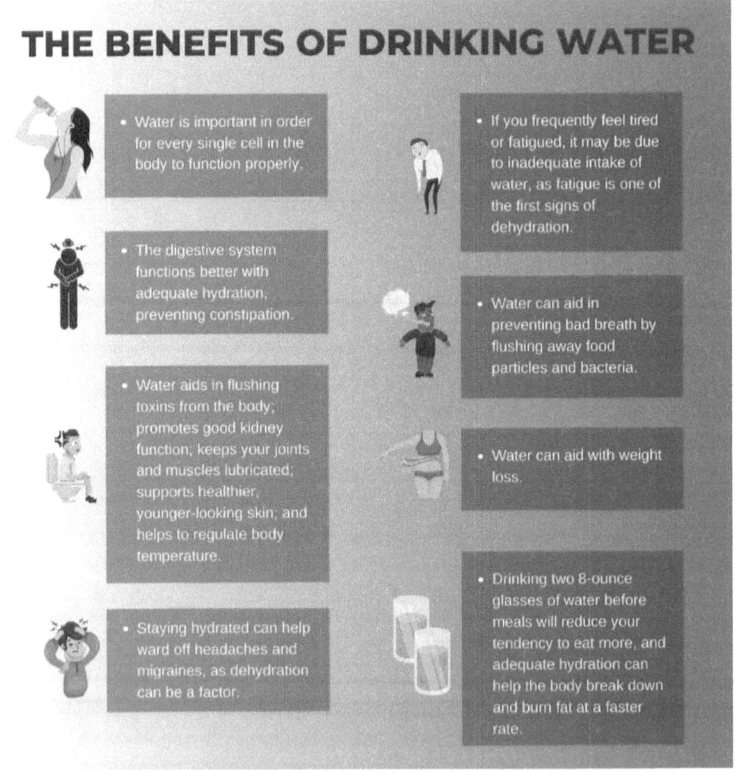

How does drinking more water help you manage blood sugar levels? When your blood sugar levels are running high, your body will try to flush excess sugar out of your blood through the urine. As a result, your body will need more fluids to rehydrate itself. Drinking water can help the body with flushing out some of the glucose in the blood.

So now that you know why water is good for you, I bet you are wondering how much should you drink, right? Would you believe me if I told you 1/2 your body weight? Let me explain.....

Let's break it down:

A 200lb person should drink 100oz of water per day. It seems like a lot but remember 60% of your body is made up of water. Keep in mind when you feel thirsty you are already dehydrated .

Here are some tips to help you drink more water.

1. Use a water bottle with a straw. It helps to consume more water faster.

2. Add non calorie flavoring to your water.

3. Drinking 1 cup of water before each meal will help fill you up and control your portions.

Chapter 5
Sleeping Beauty

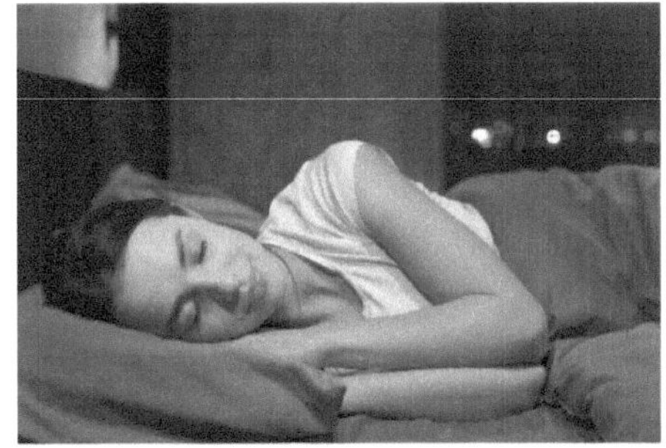

Sleeping Beauty

I'm sure you have heard that getting 8 hours of sleep is important. Sleep boosts your immune system, manages weight loss, and helps you retain memory. While lack of sleep is known to be a contributing factor for many chronic health conditions, including diabetes, heart disease, obesity, and obstructive sleep apnea.

Here are some tips to help you build better sleeping habits.

Schedule your sleep: Make an effort to go to bed and wake up at the same time every day of the week, including weekends. Doing this establishes a regular sleep-wake cycle. It may help you adopt the habit of doing the same things each night before bed, such as taking a warm bath or reading.

Avoid stimulants: Caffeine, chocolate, and nicotine can keep you awake past your bedtime. Alcohol may make you feel sleepy initially, but its effect eventually may disrupt your rest later in the night. Stay away from stimulants at least four hours before sleep.

Make your bed comfy: A number of new mattresses on the market are aimed at increasing comfort, including those that have "cooling" effects to keep a person from getting too warm while they sleep. Memory-foam mattresses conform to a person's body, providing extra shape and support. Use room-darkening shades, earplugs, or other tools that will help create a restful environment.

Relieve stress during the day: Try adopting some stress-reducing techniques before bed. Keep a journal by your bedside to write down what's bothering you. Start practicing yoga, learn to meditate, get regular massages, or take long walks.

Exercise regularly: Being physically active during the day can help you fall asleep faster at night and promotes deeper, more restful sleep. Just make sure you don't exercise too close to bedtime, since this can leave you too energized to sleep.

Use an App for sleep:
Some apps can help you sleep better.

The Sleep Genius tracks your sleep cycles and offers a progressive alarm clock to prevent sudden waking that's associated with increased tiredness.

 Other apps, like the ZZZ app, provide soft music and sounds used to encourage restful sleep.

Chapter 6
Get Moving

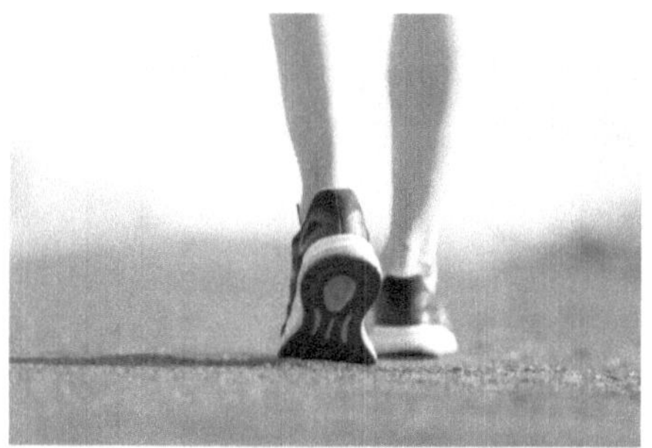

Get Moving

Ok so the last thing on the list is to get moving! A sedentary lifestyle is one of the many risk factors for type 2 diabetes. So if you are not used to being active this is one lifestyle change that will make a big difference.

Just like all the lifestyle changes here you can start off slowly and increase as your tolerance increases.

How does physical acitivy affect type 2 diabetes? Studies have shown that your insulin resistance goes down when you exercise, and your cells can use the glucose more effectively. The benefits are even greater when you incorporate both aerobic and strength training.

Additionally, there are also the traditional benefits of exercise:

Lower blood pressure
Better control of weight
Increased level of good cholesterol (HDL) Leaner,
Stronger muscles
Stronger bones
More energy
Improved mood
Better sleep
Stress management

Before starting any exercise program be sure to talk to your doctor first. Now let's talk about what kinds of exercise to do. There are three main kinds of exercise: aerobic, strength training, and flexibility. You should aim to have a good balance of all three.

Aerobic exercises include:

Walking

Jogging/Running

Sports like Tennis, Basketball, Raquetball,

Swimming

Biking

You should aim to get at least 30 minutes of aerobic exercise most days of the week. If you think that you can't find 30 minutes, you can break up the exercise into chunks— 10 minutes here and there. Build up to 30 minutes gradually.

Stretch your creativity when it comes to fitting in exercise.

Take a walk at lunch
Get the whole family out after dinner for a game of basketball
Dancing in the comfort of your own home. Walking your dog is a form of exercise Taking the stairs is exercise.
Walking from your car and into the store is exercise— so park farther away.

You need to find a way to exercise that you actually enjoy—because if it's not fun, you won't do it. It'll be harder to stay motivated, even if you know all the benefits of exercise. Consider taking group classes at the gym, or find a friend to walk or run with. Having someone else exercising with you does make it more fun and motivating.

Strength Training

Once you have been able to include aerobic activity into your days, then you can start including strength training.

Strength training gives you lean, efficient muscles, and it also helps you maintain strong, healthy bones. It's really good for you when you have type 2 diabetes because muscles use the most glucose, so if you can use them more, then you'll be better able to control your blood glucose level.

Weight training is one of the most used strength training techniques, although you can also use exercise bands or your own body weight to build up strength—think of pull-ups and push-ups.

Lifting weights for 20-30 minutes two or three times a week is sufficient to get the full benefits of strength training.

A Physical Therapist can help you choose the right exercises and amount of weight to start with to avoid injury or reinjury.

Flexibility Training

With flexibility training, you'll improve how well your muscles and joints work. Stretching before and after exercise (especially after exercise) reduces muscle soreness and actually relaxes your muscles.

Let's Review

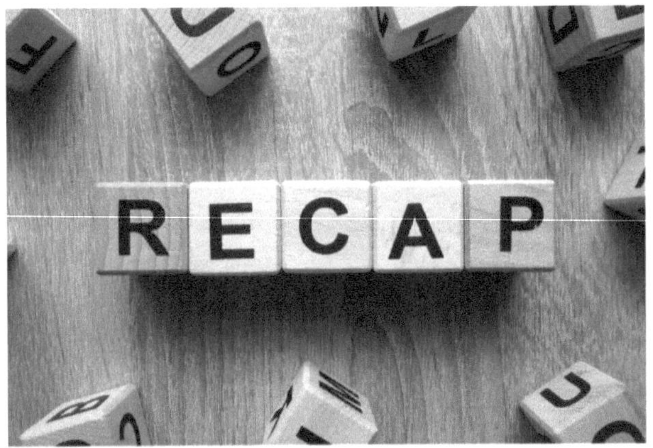

Recap

In conclusion, these lifestyle changes in small increments can help you get started on a healthier lifestyle and reducing your risks of type 2 diabetes as well as reversing it. One of the key components in my personal journey was having accountability and support.

If you would like to learn more about our diabetes program that can provide you with structured exercises, accountability, support, and nutritional ideas then feel free to reach out to talk to a Physical Therapist on our website at www.madeformotionllc.com

Resources

STRATEGY
LEARN
MEDIA
TEACH
COLLEGE
INTELLIGENCE
DISCOVER
TEACH
SKILL
DISCOVER
TEACHER
INSTRUCTION
INFORMATION
EDUCATIONAL
RESOURCES
SUCCESS
PLAN
PROJECT
GOAL
SUCCESSFUL
DISCOVER
TEACH
LEARN

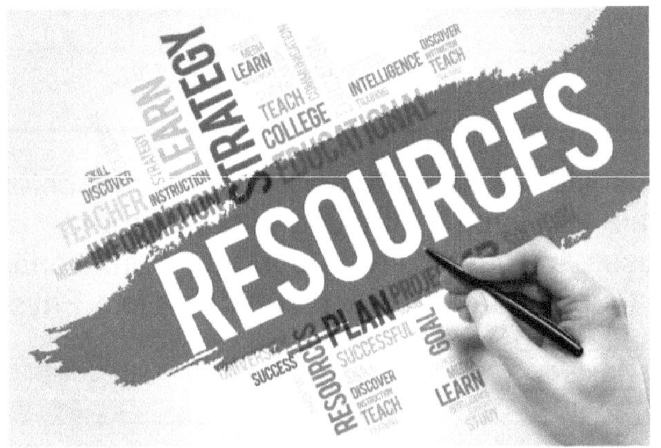

Resources

1. https://www.diabetes.co.uk/food/water-and-diabetes.html
2. Endocrineweb https://www.endocrineweb.com/conditions/type-2-diabetes/type-2-diabetes-exercise
3. Office of Women's Helath: www.womenshealth.gov
4. Centers for Disease Control and Prevention (CDC). (2017). National diabetes statistics report, 2017 (PDF, 1.4 MB).
5. Coustan, D. R. (Ed). (2013). Medical management of pregnancy complicated by diabetes. 5th edition. Alexandria, VA:
6. American Diabetes Association. (2013). Standards of medical care in diabetes — 2013. Diabetes Care, 36(Suppl. 1), S11–66.
7. National Institute of Diabetes and Digestive and Kidney Diseases. (NIDDK). (2017). Type 1 diabetes.

Contact Information

You may contact Dr. Belisa Kinnard at by emailing her at belisa@madeformotionllc.com.
We can also be reached by phone at 717-897-0874 if you would like a free phone consult.
You can visit our various platforms for more information including
Website: www.madeformotionllc.com
Facebook: www.facebook.com/madeformotionllc
Instagram: www.instagram.com/madeformotionllc

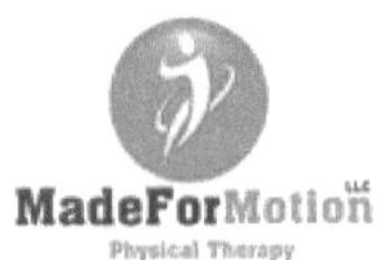